DASH Diet Slow Cooker Cookbook: The Best Dash Diet Recipes For Healthy Weight Loss

Disclaimer and Terms of Use: Effort has been made to ensure that the information in this book is accurate and complete, however, the author and the publisher do not warrant the accuracy of the information, text and graphics contained within the book due to the rapidly changing nature of science, research, known and unknown facts and internet. The Author and the publisher do not hold any responsibility for errors, omissions or contrary interpretation of the subject matter herein. This book is presented solely for motivational and informational purposes only.

Table of Contents

Wine and Tomato Chicken

Ingredients:
- 1 onion sliced
- ½ lbs. bacon
- 1 4 T minced garlic
- 1 tsp thyme
- 1 tsp fennel
- 1 tsp salt and pepper to taste
- 1 C dry white wine
- 1 can whole tomatoes
- One dozen chicken thighs, meat deboned
- ¼ C chopped parsley

Directions: Cook the bacon and crumble, or you can use bacon bits. Yu can use a few T of the bacon fat to cook the onions, stirring, add the rest of our spices, then wine, add the chicken into slow cooker then bacon shred, tomatoes, juice, and cook for about 3-4 hours in slow cooker.

Slow cooked pulled pork

Ingredients:

- 1 T olive oil
- 2 lbs. butt roast, shaved
- 3 onions, diced
- ½ C raw sugar
- 4 T minced garlic
- 1 tsp oregano
- 1 tsp salt and pepper to taste
- 1/3 C apple cider vinegar
- 1 C chili sauce
- 1 ½ tsp minced jalapeño's

Directions: You can sauté the onions and spices in a skillet ten add them to your slow cooker with 1-2 C water and your butt roast. Cook for 6-8 hours on low and shred

Moroccan Soup

Ingredients:
- 2 C chopped onions
- 2 C diced carrots
- 4 T minced garlic
- 2 tsp virgin olive oil
- 1 tsp cumin
- 1 tsp coriander
- ¼ tsp cinnamon
- 6 C chicken broth
- 2 C water
- 3 C diced cauliflower
- 1 ¾ C lentils
- 1 can diced tomatoes
- 2 T tomato paste
- 4 C shredded spinach
- ½ C fresh cilantro

Directions: Add everything into slow cooker and cook for 6-8 hours on high.

Pinto Bean stew

Ingredients:

- 1 lbs. soaked pinto beans
- 6 C water
- 1 bell pepper chopped
- Onion diced
- 1 C frozen corn
- 2 celery sticks, chopped
- 2 T minced garlic
- 2 T chili powder
- 2 T lime juice

Dumplings

- 1.2 C flour
- ½ C cornmeal
- ½ tsp cornmeal
- Salt and pepper to taste
- 2 T butter
- 1 jalapeño, chopped
- ½ C buttermilk

Directions: You will set your slow cooker on low, and add everything to the slow cooker, except for the dumpling ingredients. You will prepare those in the a bowl and add the dumplings and turn heat to high and cook for one more hour

Beefy Bean chili

Ingredients:
- 1 lbs. ground beef, cooked and strained
- 2 cans cooked beans
- 4 cans tomatoes and chilies
- 1 onion diced
- 1 T olive oil
- Salt & pepper to taste
- 2 tsp. cumin
- ¼ C chili powder
- 1 tsp sugar
- 1 T minced garlic
- 1 T cayenne pepper

Directions: Cook the onions in your skillet and add to slow cooker with remaining ingredients and set on low for about 4-6 hours

Healthy man's stew

Ingredients:
- 7 ½ chopped rutabaga
- 6 C diced carrots
- 1 C sliced celery
- 18 C water
- 2 C chickpeas
- 5 T minced garlic
- 1 T dash seasoning
- 1 C Dijon
- 1 T extra virgin olive oil
- 2 T low sodium vegetable broth
- 6 C spinach

Directions: Add everything in to your slow cooker and cook on low for about 6 hours or so, add the spinach during the last 30-45 minutes.

Tex Tortilla soup

Ingredients:
- 1 lbs. chicken tenders or bites
- 2 cans black beans
- 2 C stewed tomatoes
- 1 C salsa
- 12 oz. tomato sauce
- Tortilla chips
- 1 C shredded cheese

Directions: ad everything but the last two ingredients, and cook for about 2 hours. Cut the chicken up, and serve with the tortilla soup and cheese

Spicy Beans

Ingredients:
- 7 C water
- 2 T lime juice
- 1 T olive oil
- 2 onions diced
- 1 pepper diced
- 4 T minced garlic
- 1 can black beans, drained
- 1 T dash seasoning
- 1 T chopped chipotle
  Directions: add everything to slow cooker and set on high for 4-6 hours.

Curry Carrots

Ingredients:
- 1 T olive oil
- 1 T minced garlic
- 1 T gluten free curry powder
- 1 leek
- 6 carrots, diced
- 1 sweet potato, sliced
- ½ banana squash, peeled, sliced
- Dash seasoning to taste

Directions: add everything together in the slow cooker, and season with Dash seasoning to taste. Cook on low for about 6 hours.

Cajun character stew

Ingredients:
- 3 ½ lbs. kielbasa
- 1 onion sliced
- 2 T minced garlic
- 2 stalks celery, diced
- 1 bell pepper, diced
- 2 T flour
- 1 can diced tomatoes and chilies
- ½ T cayenne pepper
- ½ lbs. shrimp, peeled
- 2 C cut okra

Directions: Add everything to slow cooker and cook on low for 6-8 hours.

Dash Diet Breakfasts

Dash Diet Apples

Ingredients:
- ½ lbs. apples, cut up
- ¼ C raisins
- ¼ C honey
- 1 tsp cinnamon
- 6 T butter

Directions: add everything to slow cooker and with ½" water, and cook overnight or at least 8 hours.

Home Yogurt

Ingredients:
- ½ gallon 2 % milk
- ½ C plain unflavored yogurt
- ¼ C powdered milk

Directions: Add milk to slow cooker and set to high, heat the milk for about 2 hours or so, give or take, add the yogurt and powdered milk. Let sit for about 6 hours. Then you have great Greek yogurt.

Beef breakfast burritos

Ingredients:
- 1 ¼ lbs. ground beef, cooked and strained
- 12 oz. tomatoes and green chilies
- 1 onion diced
- 1 jalapeño, diced
- ½ tsp ground chipotle
- ¼ tsp cayenne pepper
- 2 T minced garlic

Directions: Add everting to slow cooker and cook for 8 hours Stir, and serve and you can add eggs as well.

Slow cooked banana bread

Ingredients:
- 1 C quinoa
- 1 C coffee mate of your preferred flavor
- ½ C 2 % milk
- 1 C water
- 2 bananas
- 2 T chopped pecans
- 3 T brown sugar
- 2 T melted butter
- 1 T vanilla extract

Directions: Mash the bananas, these need to be PAST ripe for sure, add the brown sugar and walnuts pour creamer and everything else to the slow cooker and cook for about 4 hours on low, you can add other low sodium or calorie flavorings if you would like. Serve warm

Cocoa Oatmeal

Ingredients:
- 1 C oats
- 4 C water
- 1 C coconut milk
- 1 T vanilla extract
- ¼ tsp. dash seasoning
- 1 T coconut milk
- 8-10 drops stevia

Directions: Combine the ingredients together, and cook for 1-2 hours on low and be sure that it keeps warm. You can add a few pieces or shaves of chocolate when serving.

Almond chocolate cherry Oatmeal

Ingredients:
- 5 C rolled oats
- 1 C almonds
- ½ C dried cherries
- ½ C pumpkin seeds
- ¼ C shredded coconut
- ¼ C canola oil
- ¼ C honey

Directions: Add everything to the slow cooker and cook for about an hour on high, but leave the lid off. Reduce to low adding coconuts, cherries and pumpkin seeds and cook for another 4 hours, without the kid. You need to stir often.

Gluten Free Banana Bread

Ingredients:
- 2-3 ripe bananas
- Dash diet seasoning
- Traditional banana bread ingredients
  Directions: add to slow cooker and cook for 4 hours in slow cooker, or in bread pan inside of slow cooker.

Pumpkin buns

Ingredients:
- 3 C flour
- ¼ C sugar
- 1 packet yeast
- ½ C vanilla almond milk
- ¼ C water
- ¾ C puree pumpkin
- ½ C canola oil
- 1 egg

1. Filling:
   - 1/3 C butter
   - 1/3 C brown sugar
   - 2 tsp cinnamon
   - 2 tsp nutmeg
   - 1 tsp ginger

2. Icing Ingredients:
   - 4 oz. cream cheese
   - 1 C powdered sugar
   - ½ stick low sodium butter
   - ½ tsp vanilla extract
   - ½ tsp lemon juice

Directions: Stir the flour sugar and yeast and stir or fold in almond milk, water flaxseed and eggs, along with the oil. Make dough and set with towel over it for about 45 minutes then roll into rectangular shape. Mix together the filling ingredients and "frost" with rectangular shape and roll into cinnamon bun shapes. Grease your slow cooker, and cook for about an hour on high, make the icing, and pour over cinnamon rolls

Dash Diet Fish and vegan slow cooker recipes

Loaded Baked potatoes

Ingredients:
- ½ dozen potatoes
- 2 T olive oil
- 10 oz. mushrooms, sliced
- ½ lbs. broccoli, chopped
- ½ C chicken broth
- 2/3 C unflavored yogurt

Directions: wrap the potatoes in foil and add top slow cooker, on low for about 8 hours. In a skillet add the oil and other mushrooms and sauté, then add broccoli. Split potatoes and scoop into bowl, but save the skin, add broth and yogurt and stir. Season with Dash diet seasoning to taste and stir. Divide into the potato skills and add broccoli stuffing and serve.

Shrimp Risotto

Ingredients:
- 3 C water
- 3 T lobster base
- 1 C chopped onion
- 3 T minced garlic
- I package frozen artichokes
- 1 C pear barley
- 1 lbs. prepared shrimp
- ¼ C parmesan
- 4 oz. spinach

Directions: Boil the water and add the lobster base, and keep warm but set aside. In a skillet sauté the onions and garlic, move to slow cooker and add rest of ingredients except for cheese and shrimp. You can add those in about 15 minutes before serving. Cook in slow cooker for about 3-4 hours on high. Season to taste with Dash diet seasoning.

Slow cooked tamale pie

Ingredients:
- 1 package corn meal
- 2 onion diced
- 2 C soy burger, crumbled or diced
- 1 can kidney beans
- 1 can enchilada sauce
- 1/3 C milk
- 2 T butter
- 1 egg
- ½ C shredded cheese
- 1 an chopped chilies
- ¼ C sour cream
- 4 green onions, diced

Directions: Spray the slow cooker, cook the onion over skillet on medium heat, stir and add everything to slow cooker. Add cheese and chilies last, and cook for 4 and a half hours and serve with sour cream and green onions

Veggie Slow cooked lasagna

Ingredients:
- 1 egg
- 1 container ricotta
- 1 can sliced mushrooms
- 1 zucchini sliced
- 1 can crushed tomatoes
- 1 can diced tomatoes and chilies
- 2 T minced garlic
- No bake lasagna noodles
- 2 C shredded cheese

Directions: This will be like your traditional lasagna, only dash diet friendly and made in slow cooker. Mix sauce and veggie ingredients and layer. Cook in slow cooker for about 4 hours on low.

Squash Lasagna

Ingredients:
- No bake lasagna noodles
- 2 cans pureed squash
- ½ tsp sage
- ½ C milk
- ¼ C parmesan
- ½ C parmesan
- ½ C spinach

Directions: Mix the squash, sage, and other seasonings and spinach, blend well. This will be your sauce. Layer your lasagna as usual i.e.: sauce, noodles, cheese repeat. Bake on low for 4 hours in slow cooker. Top with parmesan

Cauliflower potatoes

Ingredients:
- 1 head cauliflower
- 3 C water
- 4 T minced garlic
- 1 tsp dash diet seasoning
- 1 T butter

Directions: take head florets and add to slow cooker, add water and rest of ingredients and cook for 2-3 hours on high or 4-6 on low. You can use a potato masher or blend in mixer and add butter, chives and onions for garnishes.

Easy Saturday Goulash

Ingredients:
- 1-2 lbs. ground beef, cooked and drained
- 1 C shredded cheese
- 1 can low sodium pasta sauce
- 1 can tomatoes and chilies, low sodium
- 1 box macaroni noodles

Directions: Add everything to slow cooker and cook on low for 4-6 hours.

Dessert

Pears and caramel sauce

Ingredients:
- 1 ½ C brown sugar
- 1 T grated ginger
- 2 T unsalted butter
- 4 firm bears
- 1/8 tsp cinnamon

Directions: in your slow cooker add the sugar and butter and ginger. Add the peeled and sliced pears and add them to the sugar mix in the slow cooker. Set to high and cook for two hours you want the pears to be tender. You can keep adding the sauce over the pears and let simmer.

October Bread

Ingredients:
- ½ C oil
- ½ C sugar
- ½ C brown sugar
- 2 beaten eggs
- 1 can pumpkin
- 1 ½ C flour
- ¼ tsp Dash diet seasoning
- ½ tsp. cinnamon
- 1 tsp. baking soda

Directions: add the oil and sugars in a bowl than the eggs and pumpkin mix. Add the Rest of the dry ingredients and add to bread pan that will fit in slow cooker, before adding lid and paper towels (10 or so) to keep the lid from bubbling (keep hot air in). Cook for 2-3 hours on low.

Orange cheesecake

Ingredients:
- Graham cracker crust
- ¾ C water
- 3 T cornstarch
- 8 oz. cream cheese
- 8 oz. tofu
- 2/3 C sugar
- 2 T brown sugar
- 1 tsp vanilla extract
- Juice from one orange

Directions: add water to slow cooker and turn o high and add lid. Add cornstarch to the slow cooker and remaining ingredients to blender with water and starch, and blend until creamy add orange juice and peels, and blend another 3 seconds Pour into graham cracker crust and add to slow cooker for 3 hours on high. Than chill for a few hours before serving.

Slow Cooker Chicken

Buttermilk Chicken

Ingredients:
- 1 Roaster
- 2 C buttermilk
- ¼ C brown sugar
- 1 T paprika
- 1 tsp Dash diet seasoning

Directions: In a baggy add everything but the brown sugar and shake really well. You need to let this set in the fridge for 24 hours before cooking. Then you can add the chicken breast side down in the slow cooker with the brown sugar and cook for 7 hours on low or 4-6 hours on high.

Chicken Meatloaf

Ingredients:
- 1 lbs. ground chicken
- Onion diced
- 2 eggs
- 1 ½ C bread crumbs
- 1 T dash diet seasoning
- 1 T minced garlic
- 1 C cooked pasta
- 2 C shredded mozzarella cheese

Directions: Start with a mixing bowl and add the ingredients and cook for about 7 or 8 hours on low.

Chicken Curry Chili

Ingredients:
- 1 lbs. chicken cooked and cut up
- 1 onion sliced
- 1 zucchini, sliced
- 1 pepper, sliced
- 6 T minced garlic
- 2 cans white beans
- 2 cans diced tomatoes
- 2 T curry powder
- 1 T chili powder
- 2 T dash diet seasoning
- ½ C broth

Directions: Add everything to the slow cooker and cook for about 8 hours on low.

Chicken Noodle Soup

Ingredients:
- 1 lbs. chicken breast
- 1 can cream of chicken soup
- 1 bag frozen egg drop noodles
- Frozen carrots and celery
- 1 C chicken broth
  Directions: add everything to slow cooker and let set on low for 6-8 hours.

Peanut butter Chicken

Ingredients:
- 1 whole chicken gutted and washed
- ½ C crunchy peanut butter
- ¼ C soy sauce
- ¼ C brown sugar
- 3 T white vinegar
- 3 T water
- 2 T minced garlic

Directions: Whisk the peanut butter, soy, brown sugar, garlic and vinegar and pour over the chicken in the slow cooker. Let cook for about 6 to 8 hours. Great with rice

Green Olive chicken

Ingredients:
- 1 T butter
- 1 T olive oil
- 2 T lemon rind
- 3 T minced garlic
- ¼ C green olives, diced
- 2 T parsley
- 1 whole chicken cut up

Directions: add all the ingredients and mix well and marinade chicken. Cook in slow cooker for 6 to 8 hours. 37.

Black Bean Chili

Ingredients:
- 2 Can black beans
- 2 cans diced tomatoes
- 1 C corn
- ½ lbs. scallions, diced
- 2 T minced garlic
- 1 T chili powder
- ½ tsp Dash diet seasoning
- 1 its cocoa powder
- 8 oz. sour cream

Directions: add everything but the sour cream to the slow cooker and cook on low for 8 hours. Use the sour cream as a garnish

Jambalaya

Ingredients:
- 1 onion, diced
- 2 T minced garlic
- Celery diced
- Carrots, diced
- Red peppers diced
- 1 tomato, diced
- 1 brown rice
- 1 lbs. ground sausage
- 1 tsp hot sauce
- 1 T dash diet seasoning
- 1 lbs. shrimp, prepared

Directions: Add everything to the slow cooker and let cook for about 8 hour or so ON low, add the shrimp and rice for the last hour of cooking if needed.

Dumplings

Ingredients:
- 1 lbs. chicken breast, cut up
- 2 cans low sodium chicken stock
- 1 container mixed vegetables
- 1 onion, diced
- 1 ½ bisquick
- ½ C 2 % milk

Directions: Add the first four ingredients together and cook for 2 ½ hour on high. Add the milk and bisquick in a bowl and add drops in to the slow cooker and cook for one more hour.

No Salt Sweet & sour chicken

Ingredients:
- 1 can pineapple, slices
- ¼ C brown sugar
- ¼ C apple cider vinegar
- 2 T soy
- 2 T cornstarch
- 1 T minced garlic
- 2 lbs. chicken breasts, chopped
- 1 bell pepper chopped
- 1 onion chopped
- ½ C sliced carrots

Directions: Save the pineapple juice from pan, add the everything into slow cooker but the pineapple and cook for about 6 hours. Serve with the pineapple and steamed rice or noodles.

BBQ Beef meat

Ingredients:
- ½ Tomato sauce
- ½ C apple juice
- 2 T maple juice
- 1 T flour
- 2 tsp red pepper flakes
- 1 T dash diet low sodium seasoning
- 2 lbs. top round roast
- 2 sliced sweet onions, sliced and diced

Directions: Add everything to the slow cooker and cook for 8-10 hours on low shred the meat as it gets tender.

Ingredients:
- 3 T flour
- 2 T brown sugar
- 2 T apple cider vinegar
- 1 C diced tomatoes
- ¼ T minced garlic
- 2 C shredded cabbage
- 1-3 lbs. beef short ribs

Directions: Add the sugar and flour together and add the wine and vinegar and whisk into the mixture. Add the rest of the ingredients, but add the ribs last. Fold those in and cook for 8 hours on low.

Low Sodium Pot roast

Ingredients:
- ½ Flour
- 2-3 lbs. beef roast
- 1 bag frozen vegetables
- 1 diced onion
- 1 T dash diet seasoning
- 1 can beef broth

Directions: Add everything together and cook for about 8 hours on low.

Chicken and Rice

Ingredients:
- Diced carrots
- Sliced leeks
- 1 C uncooked rice
- 1 lbs. chicken breasts
- 1 tsp thyme
- ½ tsp rosemary
- 4 C chicken broth
- 1 can cream of chicken soup
- 1 C chopped onion
- 1 T minced garlic

Directions: add everything together and cook in slow cooker for about 6-8 hours.

Chicken and Salsa

Ingredients:
- 2-4 lbs. chicken breast
- 2 C salsa
- 1 can corn
- 1 can black beans
- 1 onion, diced
- 1 red pepper, chopped

Directions: add the chicken to the slow cooker first, and add vegetables, then salsa last. Cook for 4-6 hours on low.

Cabbage and sausage

Ingredients:
- 1-2 cabbage heads, shredded or sliced
- 1 onion, sliced
- 1 package sausage links
- ½ lbs. small red potatoes
- 1 C apple juice
- 1 T mustard
- 1 T cider vinegar
- 1 T brown sugar
- 1 tsp caraway seed

Directions: Start with the cabbage on the bottom, then onion, and sausage, sliced or diced. Whisk the other ingredients, and add to the slow cooker and cook on low for 6-8 hours.

Ham and Peas

Ingredients:
- 1 package diced ham
- 2 cans peas
- 1 C carrots, sliced
- 8 C water
- 1 onion diced
- Dash diet seasoning to taste

Directions: add everything to slow cooker and cook on low for about 6 hours or high for 4 hours.

Hot Green Soup

Ingredients:
- 1 lbs. ground beef, cooked and strained
- 1 onion, diced
- 2 C diced tomatoes and chilies
- 2 peppers, diced
- 2 C tomato sauce
- 2 C water
- 1 T beef granules
- 1 C uncooked rice

Directions: Add everything in slow cooker, and cook for 4-6 hours, Add rice for the last 3—45 minutes.

Chicken stroganoff and noodles

Ingredients:
- 1 lbs. chicken breasts
- 1 C cream of mushroom soup
- 1 container low fat sour cream
- 1 envelope dried onion soup

Directions: add everything to slow cooker and cook on low for 6 hours, serve with cooked white rice or egg noodles

Low Sodium Dash Diet spaghetti Sauce

Ingredients:

- 1 C vegetable protein
- 1 C diced tomatoes
- 2 tomatoes chopped
- 1 tsp dash diet seasoning
- 1 green pepper shredded or sliced in thin pieces
- 2 tsp sugar
- ¼ tsp oregano
- ¼ tsp basil
- ¼ tsp minced garlic

Directions: add everything to slow cooker on low and simmer or cook on LOW for 8-10 hours